Sirtfood D

CW00460885

Uncover your happy Weight Despite Menopause and Hormonal Imbalance

Jane Harris

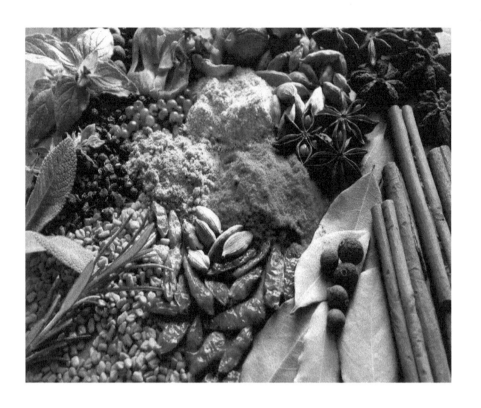

Sommario

WHAT IS THE SIRTFOOD DIET?

Sirtuins are a group of proteins that manage cell wellbeing. Sirtuins assume a key job in controlling cell homeostasis.

In the cells, numerous pieces are taking a shot at different undertakings with an extreme objective, as well: remain sound and capacity proficiently for whatever length of time that conceivable. Similarly, as needs in the organization change, because of different inside and outer variables, so do needs in the cells. Somebody needs to run the workplace, directing what completes when, who will do it and when to switch course.

NAD+ is essential to cell digestion and many other organic procedures. If sirtuins are an organization's CEO, at that point, NAD+ is the cash that pays the pay of the CEO and workers, all while keeping the lights on and the workplace space lease paid. An organization, and the body, can't work without it.

Protein may seem like dietary protein — what's found in beans and meats and well, protein shakes — yet for this situation we're discussing atoms called proteins, which work all through the body's phones in various capacities.

Consider proteins the divisions at an organization, everyone concentrating without anyone else explicit capacity while planning with different offices.

Acetyl groups control explicit responses. They're physical labels on proteins that different proteins perceive will respond with them. If proteins are the branches of the cell and DNA are the CEO, the acetyl groups are the accessibility status of every division head. For instance, if a protein is accessible, at that point the sirtuins can work with it to get something going; similarly, as the CEO can work with an accessible division head to get something going.

Sirtuins work with acetyl groups by doing what's called deacetylation. One way that sirtuins work is by evacuating acetyl gatherings deacetylation organic proteins, for example, histones. The histone is an enormous cumbersome protein that the DNA folds itself over. This loosened up chromatin implies the DNA is being translated, a fundamental procedure.

We've just thought about sirtuins for around 20 years, and their essential capacity was found during the 1990s. From that point forward, specialists have rushed to examine them, recognizing their significance while likewise bringing up issues about what else we can find out about them.

In 1991, Elysium fellow benefactor and MIT scientist Leonard Guarantee, along with graduate understudies Nick Austria and Brian Kennedy, directed tests to all the more likely see how yeast matured. By some coincidence, Austria attempted to develop societies of different yeast strains from tests he had put away in his ice chest for quite a long time, which made an unpleasant situation for the strains.

This is the place acetyl groups become possibly the most important factor. It was their first idea that SIR2 may be a deacetylation protein — which means it expelled those acetyl gatherings — from different atoms, however, nobody knew whether this was valid since all endeavors to show this movement in a test tube demonstrated negative.

In Guarantee's very own words: "Without NAD+, SIR2 sirts idle. That was the basic finding on the circular segment of sirtuins science."

Ecological factors significantly influence the destiny of living beings and sustenance is one of the most persuasive variables. These days life span is a significant objective of medicinal science and has consistently been a fabrication for the individual since antiquated occasions. Specifically, endeavors are planned for accomplishing effective maturing, to be a long life without genuine ailments, with a decent degree of physical and mental autonomy and satisfactory social connections.

Gathering information unmistakably exhibits that it is conceivable to impact the indications of maturing. Without a doubt, wholesome mediations can advance wellbeing and life span. A tribute must be given to Ansel Keys, who was the first to give strong logical proof about the job of sustenance in the wellbeing/sickness balance at the populace level, explicitly in connection to cardiovascular illness, still the main source of death overall. It is commonly valued that the sort of diet can significantly impact the quality and amount of life and the Mediterranean eating regimen is paradigmatic of an advantageous

dietary example. The developing cognizance of the useful impacts of a particular dietary example on wellbeing and life span in the second half of the remaining century produced a ground-breaking push toward structuring eating fewer carbs that could diminish the danger of constant maladies, subsequently bringing about solid maturing. Subsequently, during the 1990s the Dietary Approaches to Stop Hypertension Dash diet was contrived to assess whether it was conceivable to treat hypertension not pharmacologically. To be sure, the DASH diet was very like the Mediterranean Diet, being wealthy in foods grown from the ground, entire grains, and strands, while poor in creature soaked fats and cholesterol. The awesome news leaving the investigation was that not exclusively did the DASH diet lower circulatory strain, however, it additionally diminished the danger of cardiovascular infection, type 2 diabetes, a few sorts of malignant growth, and other maturing related maladies.

To additionally improve the medical advantages of plant nourishment rich, creature fat-terrible eating routines, especially in people with hypercholesterolemia, the Portfolio Diet was planned. This eating regimen, other than being to a great extent veggielover,with just limited quantities of soaked fats, prescribes likewise a high admission of utilitarian nourishments, including thick filaments, plant stools, soy proteins, and almonds. Curiously, members on the Portfolio Diet displayed a decrease of coronary illness chance related to lower plasma cholesterol in contrast with members on a sound, for the most part, vegan diet.

Additionally, the measure of ingested nourishment has been pulling in lightof a legitimate concern for mainstream researchers as a potential modifier of the harmony among wellbeing and infection in a wide range of living species.

Specifically, calorie limitation CR has been exhibited to be a rising healthful intercession that animates the counter maturing instruments in the body.

In this way, the eating routine of the individuals living on the Japanese island of Okinawa has been widely broken down because these islanders are notable for their life span and expanded wellbeing range, bringing about the best recurrence of centenarians on the planet. Interestingly, the customary Okinawan diet came about to be fundamentally the same as the Mediterranean Diet and the DASH diet regarding nourishment types. Be that as it may, the vitality admission of Okinawans, at the hour of the underlying logical perceptions, was about 20% lower than the normal vitality admission of the Japanese, along these lines deciding an average state of CR.

Singer Adele has confirmed that she has lost 30 kilos in just one year. The secret? It's all thanks to the Sirtfood Diet. It was revealed by the singer herself through international media, such as the Daily Mail and the New York Post.

The Sirtfood Diet is not the classic fasting diet: Adele is the living proof of this, given the splendid shape in which was at her appointments with her fans.

It is, in fact, a diet that leaves room for both cheese and red wine as well as chocolate, in the right proportions, and of course under the supervision of a specialist doctor, who knows how to evaluate your health and recommend the most suitable diet to lose weight safely.

Many were the media that underlined the substantial weight loss of the singer Adele who admitted how the decision to lose weight did not depend on the acceptance of her as much as the difficulty of using her voice to the fullest.

Adele praised the Sirtfood Diet, which made her lose 30 kilos without much effort although, in reality, she admitted via Instagram that she had never struggled as much in physical activity as when preparing for her tour. She also said that the beauty of Sirtfoods is that many of them are already on our table every day. They are accessible and can be easily integrated into our diet.

PHASES OF THE SIRTFOOD DIET

The diet is mainly divided into two phases: the first lasts one week and the other lasts 14 days.

Phase 1 (The Most Effective): Three Kilos in Seven Days

It is the "supersonic" phase: the calorie restriction is combined with a diet rich in Sirt foods. The novelty compared to other diets is that it fattens and fattens the muscles. Two different moments. Days 1-3 are the most intense, and during this time you can consume a maximum of one thousand calories per day. You must consume 3 Sirt green juices and a solid meal.

On days 4-7 assigned the intake of one thousand five hundred calories daily.

You have to take two green Sirt juices and two solid meals. Phase 1 is the most intense, in which the best results are seen and which allows you to lose up to 3.5 kilos.

The maximum of calories consumed during the first 3 days is 1000, while from the fourth to the seventh one reaches 1500 calories per day.

The menu to follow includes a "fixed" part, the one relating to green juice created by nutritionists that helps to moderate the appetite of the brain, and one that varies daily.

The green juice recipe is simple and includes all-natural products: 75 g of curly kale, 30 g of arugula and 5 g of parsley must be centrifuged, together with 150 g of green celery with the leaves and 1/2 green apple, grated.

Everything must be completed with half a squeezed lemon and half a teaspoon of Matcha tea.

Here is more in detail the program of the first week:

Monday - Wednesday: 3 Sirt green juices to be taken on waking up, midmorning and mid-afternoon; 1 solid meal of animal or vegan protein (for example, turkey escalope or buckwheat noodles with tofu) accompanied by vegetables, always ending with 15-20 g of 85% dark chocolate.

Thursday - Sunday: 2 Sirt green juices and 2 solid meals, remembering to always vary the main course chosen, from salmon fillet to vegetable tabbouleh to buckwheat spaghetti with celery and kale.

Phase 2 (Maintenance), For 14 Days

Every day, for 14 days, you will eat three balanced meals, chock full of Sirt foods, drink a Sirt green juice, and consume 1-2 Sirt snacks. Green juice should be taken in the morning as soon as you wake up or at least 30 minutes before breakfast, or mid-morning. The evening meal must be eaten by 7 pm.

Phase 2 is the maintenance phase. During this period the goal is the consolidation of the weight loss, although the possibility of losing weight is not excluded. To do all this, just feed on the exceptional foods rich in sirtuins.

It lasts 14 days, it is less restrictive than the first and provides for sirt foods at will: 3 solid meals plus two juices. The important thing is that they are balanced.

The positive aspects of this diet are:

One is the fact that the calorie limit is indicative and not a goal to be achieved. Another advantage is that the dishes on offer are very satisfying.

This way you won't have the hunger attacks typical of other diets. The caloric restriction of the diet even in the most intensive phase is not drastic and Sirt foods have a satiating effect, which prevents us from getting hungry at meals.

And then?

As already explained in the introduction, the Sirtfood diet cannot (and must not) continue indefinitely and for a very long time. Rather, it must be done in cycles, once, two, or three times a year. However, the sirt "lifestyle" can continue even after completing the phase.

Sirt foods can be eaten all year round, continuing to speed up the metabolism.

However, this should not be combined with a very strong calorie restriction, but only avoid eating unhealthy foods, such as fried, sweet, or unsaturated fats. Your persistence will make the difference between success and failure, remember: this is not a shot, but a marathon!

Sirt cycles are simply a boost, a powerful weapon in your arsenal that you can use twice a year (depending on your body of course), but you can have a healthy lifestyle all year round, perhaps combined with regular physical exercise.

Phase 3 (Make the Sirt Food Diet For Life)

For 1 week, the participants followed the diet and exercised daily. At the end of the week, participants lost an average of 7 pounds (3.2 kg) and maintained or even gained muscle mass.

Yet, these results are hardly surprising. Restricting your calorie intake to 1,000 calories and exercising at the same time will nearly always cause weight loss.

Regardless, this kind of quick weight loss is neither genuine nor long-lasting, and this study did not follow participants after the first week to see if they gained any of the weight back, which is typically the case.

When your body is energy-deprived, it uses up its emergency energy stores, or glycogen, in addition to burning fat and muscle.

Each molecule of glycogen requires 3–4 molecules of water to be stored.

When your body uses up glycogen, it gets rid of this water as well. It's known as "water weight."

In the first week of extreme calorie restriction, only about one-third of the weight loss comes from fat, while the other two-thirds come from water, muscle, and glycogen As soon as your calorie intake increases, your body replenishes its glycogen stores, and the weight comes right back.

Unfortunately, this type of calorie restriction can also cause your body to lower its metabolic rate, causing you to need even fewer calories per day for energy than before.

This diet may likely help you lose a few pounds in the beginning, but it'll likely come back as soon as the diet is over.

As far as preventing disease, 3 weeks is probably not long enough to have any measurable long-term impact.

On the other hand, adding Sirtfoods to your regular diet over the long term may very well be a good idea. But in that case, you might as well skip the diet and start doing that now.

The Best 20 Sirtfoods
Arugula

This green salad leaf (also known as rucola) is very common in the Mediterranean diet. It is not too popular in the US food culture, and it is considered an absolute arrogance to have it on your plate. However, we are not talking about a leaf covered in gold or silver; we are talking about a green salad leaf with a peppery taste that can be used for digestive and diuretic purposes.

During the time of ancient Rome and in the middle Ages, this leaf was known to have aphrodisiac properties. However, there is a lot more to this miracle leaf. It has nutrients like quercetin and kaempferol capable of activating sirtuins. This combination is said to have very positive effects on the skin as it can moisturize and improve collagen synthesis. So why not have this leaf in your salad and add some extra olive oil on it, making it a powerful Sirtfood duo? As you can see, it has many positive effects on your body.

Buckwheat

This is one of the best sources for rutin, a sirtuin-activator nutrient. However, this crop is also amazing for ecological and sustainable farming, as it can improve the quality of the soil and prevent weed growth. However, probably the most interesting part about buckwheat is that it is a fruit seed, kind of like rhubarb, so it is not a grain at all. It is not a coincidence at all that buckwheat has more protein than any grain known to man, so it fits perfectly in your Sirtfood diet. For every person trying to avoid gluten, this can be the ideal food. It is the ideal alternative for grains.

Capers

Some of you may not be too familiar with capers. If you have not had the chance to taste them, you should. They are those dark-green salty things you can see sometimes on top of a pizza.

Unfortunately, capers are not very used in a standard diet (it is very overlooked and underrated), but those who never had the chance to try capers do not know what they are missing. We are talking about the flower buds of the caper bush, a plant growing abundantly in the Mediterranean region. It is usually handpicked and preserved, and it has some interesting antidiabetic, anti-inflammatory, antimicrobial, antiviral, and immunomodulatory properties. Moreover, it has been used in medicine all around the Mediterranean area.

Celery

This is a plant used for thousands of years, as in ancient Egypt, people were already aware of it and its properties. Back then, it was considered a medicinal plant that can be used for detoxing, cleansing and preventing diseases.

Therefore, celery consumption is very good for your gut, kidney, and liver. When it was growing wildly in ancient times, it had a strong bitter flavor. However, ever since its domestication in the 17th century, celery has become a bit sweeter, and now it can be used in salads.

Chilies

This veggie should be in your diet whether you like eating spicy food or not.

It contains capsaicin, and this substance makes us savor it even more.

Consuming chilies is great for activating sirtuins and it speeds up your metabolism. In fact, the spicier the chili is, the more powerful it is when it comes to activating sirtuins. You probably heard that people eating spicy food three or four times per week have a 14 percent lower death rate compared to people who eat them less than once a week. Now, this does not mean that you have to go for the hottest chilies you can find, especially if you are not a spicy food enthusiast. Take it easy at the beginning.

Cocoa

The Aztecs and Mayans considered Cocoa sacred, and it was a food type reserved only for the warriors or the elite. It was often used as a currency, as people were aware of its value.

Although back then it was mostly used as a drink, you do not have to dilute it with milk or water to reap the full benefits of it. The best way to consume cocoa is by eating dark chocolate (with at least 85 percent solid cocoa).

However, this also depends on how the chocolate is made, as this product is usually treated with an alkalizing agent, which is known to lower the acidity of the chocolate and give a darker color. This substance is also known to reduce the sirtuin-activating flavanols.

Coffee

This is a drink enjoyed by most adults out there, and it is considered indispensable by most of them. We even believe that we can function without a cup of coffee to start within the morning. Obviously, that is not true, but we can honestly believe that coffee significantly improves our productivity and our daily activities. Caffeine acid is a nutrient known to activate sirtuins, so there is more to drinking coffee than a popular and very pleasant social activity.

Extra Virgin Olive Oil

This oil is perhaps the healthiest form of fats you can think of, and it is not missing from any salad in the Mediterranean diet. The health benefits of consuming this oil are countless. It prevents and fights against diabetes, different types of cancer, osteoporosis, and many more. Besides, EVO oil can be associated with increased longevity, as it also has anti-aging effects. You can easily find this type of oil in most supermarkets, so you do not have any excuse to exclude it from your Sirtfood diet. This oil has the right nutrients to activate the sirtuin gene in your body.

Garlic

I do not know about you people, but I am simply in love with garlic. I am sure I am not the only one. Forget about the smell it leaves behind. Enjoy the great taste it offers. I would have garlic with any meal. Of course, this may not fit with our busy lifestyle, as it is not recommended to have it before a meeting, but you can enjoy it for dinner or at home. However, there is more to the consumption of garlic. As you probably know, it has an antifungal and antibiotic effect and has been successfully used to treat stomach ulcers. Also,it can be used to remove waste products from your body.

Green Tea

In some cultures, drinking tea is as popular as drinking coffee, but what if you find the tea assortment that works best for you. You can indeed have tea from various medicinal plants, and they all have positive effects on your health. However, most of these plants are focused on preventing or fighting a specific disease. Have you ever thought about drinking tea for your well-being or to feel great? Well, this is what green tea is for. First appeared in Asia, green tea has become very popular in Western culture. It has plenty of antioxidants. It can be used for detox, and it speeds up your metabolism.

Kale

You can never go wrong with some leafy greens, and this is applicable for kale as well. Perhaps not many of you have tried it before, but it is totally worth it. Over the last few years, kale has gained a lot of popularity and appreciation from both nutritionists and consumers, and they have all the reasons to like and appreciate it.

Medjool Dates

If you have the chance to go to any country in the Middle East or the Arabian Peninsula, you will find that dates are a very common snack. Dehydrated, covered in chocolate, or a fresher form, dates are perhaps the most common snack you can find over there.

Parsley

The parsley leaves are extremely frequent in recipes, so it is not missing from the Sirtfood diet. You can chop them and toss them in your meal or use a sprig for decorative purposes. But parsley is not for decorating your plate, as you are not trying to impress a jury of famous chefs. This is an underrated plant.

Red Endive

This vegetable is one of the latest discoveries in the world of plants. How come? It was discovered by accident in 1830 when a Belgian farmer who stored chicory roots in his cellar, forgot about them and discovered them with white leaves that happened to be crunchy, tender, and delicious.

Red Onions

If you are only eating onions as O-rings with your burger, then you had better rethink the way you consume this incredible vegetable. This type of onion has a sweeter taste (compared to yellow onion). It has plenty of antioxidants, and it is known to fight against inflammation, heart diseases, and diabetes.

Red Wine

The Mediterranean diet encourages the consumption of red wine, and there are plenty of reasons why you should consider the moderate consumption of it. We are not going to talk about the effects it has on your blood, blood sugar level, and so on. Not even about how moderate consumption can decrease the death rates by heart disease. Alternatively, about how red wine can prevent common colds and cavities (yes, it can even improve your oral health). Red wines like

Merlot, Cabernet Sauvignon, or Pinot Noir have an incredible concentration of polyphenol to activate your sirtuins.

Soy

There is a completely food-processing industry behind soy, as it is used to create food products for vegetarians. However, let us face it — drinking soymilk will not activate your sirtuins. Industrially processed food is not very recommended for your health, so it should be excluded from your Sirtfood diet. In natural form, soy contains formononetin and daidzein, two great sirtuin-activating nutrients.

Strawberries

Of all the fruits out there, strawberries are among the ones with the most health benefits. Yes, they are sweet, but they happen to have a very high concentration of fisetin, a nutrient that can activate sirtuins. What is very confusing is that strawberries are known to prevent heart diseases, diabetes, cancer, osteoporosis, and Alzheimer's

disease. They are even associated with healthy aging. Although they are sweet, 3½ ounces of strawberries only contain a teaspoon of sugar.

Turmeric

You are probably familiar with the effects ginger has on your overall health, but you do not know what turmeric can do for you. This plant is related to ginger, and it is very appreciated throughout Asia for medical and culinary reasons. India is responsible for 80 percent of the whole turmeric on the planet, and some nutritionists refer to it as the "golden spice" or "India's gold." Why is that? Because it contains curcumin, a very rare sirtuinactivating nutrient.

Walnuts

As it happens, the walnut tree is the oldest food tree known to humans, as it was discovered around 7,000 BCE. Its original location was in ancient Persia (modern-day Iran), and now this tree is spread all around the world, as it can easily adapt to different climates of the globe. In the United States, walnuts are a success story. California is the biggest producer of walnuts in the United States, responsible for 99 percent of the US commercial supply and three-quarters of the walnut trade worldwide.

FAQ

Can Children Eat Sirtfoods?

There are powerful Sirtfoods, most of which are safe for children. Obviously, children should avoid wine, coffee, and other highly caffeinated foods, such as matcha. On the other hand, children can enjoy sirtuin-rich foods such as cabbage, eggplant, blueberries, and dates with their regular balanced diet.

Yet, while children can enjoy most sirtuin-rich foods, that is not the same as to say that they can practice the Sirt diet. This diet plan is not designed for children, and it does not fit the needs of their growing bodies. Practicing this diet plan could not only negatively affect them physically, but it could damage their mental health for years to come. Anyone can develop an eating disorder, but it is especially true for children. If you want your child to eat

well, ensure they eat a wide range of foods, as recommended by their doctor, and you can simply include an abundance of sirtuin-rich foods into what they are already eating. Leave the focus on eating healthfully and not losing weight. Even if your child's doctor does want them to lose weight, you don't need to make the child aware of this fact. You can help guide them along with a healthy lifestyle, teaching them how to eat well and stay active through sports and play, and the weight will come off naturally without placing an

unneeded burden on their small shoulders.

For similar reasons, you can include Sirtfoods in a balanced diet while pregnant, but you should avoid practicing the Sirt diet when you are pregnant. It doesn't contain the nutrition requirements for either a pregnant woman or a growing baby. Save the diet for after you have delivered a healthy baby, and both you and your child will be healthy and happy.

Can I Exercise During Phase One?

If you use exercise during either phase one or two, you can increase weight loss and health benefits. While you shouldn't work at pushing the limits during phase one, you can continue your normal workout routine and physical activity. It is important to stay within your active comfort zone during this time, as physical exertion more than you are accustomed to will be especially difficult while you are restricting your calories. It will not only wear you out, but it can also make you dizzy, more prone to injury, and physically and mentally exhausted. This is a common symptom whenever a person pushes their limits while restricting calories, but it is something you should avoid.

If you are used to doing yoga and a spin class a few times a week, keep it up!

If you are used to running a few miles a day, have at it! Do what you andbyour body are comfortable with, and as your doctor advises, and you should be fine.

I'm Already Thin. Can I Still Follow the Diet?

Whether or not you can follow the first phase of the Sirt diet will depend on just how thin you already are. While a person who is overweight or well within a healthy weight can practice the first phase, nobody who is clinically underweight should. You can know whether or not you are underweighting by calculating your Body Mass Index, or BMI. You can find many BMI calculators online, and if yours is at nineteen points or below, you should avoid the first phase. It is always a good idea to ask your doctor both if it is safe for you to lose weight, and if the Sirt diet is safe for your individual

condition. While the Sirt diet may generally be safe, for people with certain illnesses, it may not be the case.

While it is understandable to desire to be even more thin, even if you already are thin, pushing yourself past the point of being underweight is incredibly unhealthy, both physically and mentally. This fits into the category of disordered eating and can cause you a lot of harm.

Some of the side effects of pushing your body to extreme weight loss include bone loss and osteoporosis, lowered immune system, fertility problems, and an increased risk of disease. If you want to benefit from the health of the Sirt diet and are underweight, instead consume, however many calories, your doctor recommends, along with plenty of Sirtfoods. This will ensure you maintain a healthy weight while also receiving the benefits that sirtuins have to offer.

If you are thin, but still at a BMI of twenty to twenty-five, then you should be safe beginning the Sirt diet, unless otherwise instructed by your doctor.

Can You Eat Meat and Dairy On The Sirtfood Diet?

In many recipes, we choose to use Sirtfood sources of protein, such as soy, walnuts, and buckwheat. However, this does not mean that you aren't allowed to enjoy meat on the Sirt diet. Sure, it's easy to enjoy a vegan or vegetarian Sirt diet, but if you love your sources of meat, then you don't have to give them up. Protein is an essential aspect of the Sirt diet to preserve muscle tone, and whether you consume only plant-based proteins or a mixture of plant and animal-based proteins is completely up to you. And, just as you can enjoy meat, you can also enjoy moderate consumption of dairy.

Some meats can actually help you better utilize the Sirtfoods you eat. This is because the amino acid leucine can enhance the effect of Sirtfoods. You can find this amino acid in chicken, beef, pork, fish, eggs, dairy, and tofu.

Can I Drink Red Wine during Phase One?

As your calories will be so limited during the first phase, it is not recommended to drink alcohol during this phase. However, you can enjoy it in moderation during phase two and the maintenance phase.

SIRTFOOD FOR BUILDING MUSCLE

Sirtuins are a group of proteins with different effects. Sirt-1 is the protein responsible for causing the body to burn fat rather than muscle for energy, which is obviously a miracle for weight loss. Another useful aspect of Sirt-1 is its ability to improve skeletal muscle.

Skeletal muscle is all the muscles you voluntarily control, such as the muscles in your limbs, back, shoulders, and so on. There are two other types, cardiac muscle is what the heart is formed of, whilst smooth muscle is your involuntary muscles – which includes muscles around your blood vessels, face, and various parts of organs and other tissues.

Skeletal muscle is separated into two different groups, the blandly named type-1, and type-2. Type 1 muscle is effective at continued, sustained activity whereas type-2 muscle is effective at short, intense periods of activity. So, for example, you would predominantly use type-1 muscles for jogging, but type-2 muscles for sprinting.

Sirt-1 protects the type-1 muscles, but not the type-2 muscle, which is still broken down for energy. Therefore, holistic muscle mass drops when fasting, even though type-1 skeletal muscle mass increases.

Sirt-1 also influences how the muscles actually work. Sirt-1 is produced by the muscle cells, but the ability to produce Sirt-1 decreases as the muscle ages. As a result, muscle is harder to build as you age and doesn't grow as fast in response to exercise. A lack of sirt-1 also causes the muscles to become tired quicker and gradually decline over time.

When you start to consider these effects of Sirt-1, you can start to form a picture of why fasting helps keep the body supple. Fasting releases Sirt-1, which in turn helps skeletal muscle grow and stay in good shape. Sirt-1 is also released by consuming sirtuin activators, giving the Sirtfood diet its muscle retaining power.

Who Should Try the Sirtfood Diet?

The Sirtfood diet is suitable for individuals who:

- Are overweight or obese
- Want to maintain his/her weight
- Needs to have a "detox" and flush away the toxins from the body
- Have failed to lose weight using different diet techniques

- Want not only to lose weight but also build muscle
- Want a healthier lifestyle and to achieve optimal health

Health Risks for Overweight and Obesity

Type 2 Diabetes - This disease occurs when the blood sugar level becomes higher than normal. According to studies, about 80% of individuals afflicted with Type 2 diabetes are overweight. What makes diabetes a killer disease is that it is a major cause of stroke, heart disease, kidney diseases, amputation, and even blindness.

Sleep Apnea - This is when an individual pauses in breathing while sleeping. Being overweight or obese is a risk factor. Why?

This is because of the fats stored in the neck area making the air pathway smaller. Besides, the fat could also cause inflammation.

Sleep apnea should not be taken lightly because it can also result in heart failure.

High Blood Pressure - Also known as hypertension, this condition refers to a state when your systolic blood pressure (usually above 140) is consistently higher than your diastolic blood pressure (usually about 90). How does being overweight make you a high risk for hypertension? Generally, a larger body size will increase your blood pressure so that your heart will have to work harder to produce the necessary supply of blood to all cells. Also, your excess body fats can damage your kidneys (your kidney helps your body regulate blood pressure). High blood pressure can result in kidney failure, heart diseases, and stroke.

Fatty Liver Disease - This is when there is a build-up of fat around the liver which can cause damage.

Reproductive issues - Menstrual issues and ultimately infertility are some of the issues experienced by overweight women.

Cancer - If you are obese or overweight, then the risk of acquiring cancer of the breast, gallbladder, colon, and endometrial increases.

These are only some of the diseases associated with being overweight. Not to mention the social, emotional, and psychological impact of the extra weight.

It stresses the importance of finding the right "strategy" to lose those excess pounds. And we have the perfect solution –the Sirtfood diet.

Are You Familiar with These Scenarios?

You know that you have overindulged during the holidays, but as you weigh yourself, you literally would want to shave all the extra pounds because you did not expect to have gained that much weight!

There is an upcoming wedding event, and you need to lose those extra pounds to fit into your gown/suit. There is no way that you are going to lose that much weight in 2 months!

You know that you are overweight and just plain unhealthy. You have already tried many diets but to no avail. Either you feel that those diets are too restrictive, there is an adverse health effect, and the diet is too expensive to maintain. Speaking of maintenance, you are having a hard time keeping off the little weight that you have managed to lose!

You are getting older and you start to notice that aside from having a hard time dealing with hangovers and late-night parties, losing and maintaining weight is not that easy as it used to be. You are not a big fan of eliminating numerous food groups and doing rigorous exercise.

You have probably heard these scenarios too many times before and you have probably experienced one or two, or you are in one of these scenarios right now. Being overweight or obese is actually one of the most common health problems around the world. According to the World Health Organization (WHO), being overweight is when your BMI is equal to or greater than 25 while being obese is when your BMI is equal to or greater than 30.

In the 2014 data from WHO, worldwide obesity has more than doubled since 1980, and more than 1.9 billion adults are overweight; and it would safe to conclude that after two years that that number has already increased significantly.

Health experts agree that this is a very alarming rate, but the good news is, obesity or having excess weight is preventable and reversible.

As you will notice, most of these scenarios are focused on aesthetics—looking good and feeling more confident about your body, but what I would like to stress is the ill-effects of every extra bulge or pound that we carry. The possible health illnesses associated with being overweight are the primary reason why you need to try the revolutionary SirtFood diet.

BENEFITS OF SIRTFOOD DIET

Fight Fat

The problem with most diets is that once you stop eating them, you will return to your unhealthy eating habits and regain the weight that you are losing. This has happened to many people after stopping their diet. The real challenge is maintaining your weight if you are satisfied with your weight loss so far.

The Sirtfood diet is also known to control appetite and I don't mean the mind control that fasting encourages. The increase in leptin satisfies us as it reduces our hunger. Makes sense right? Leptin is important as it is the hormone responsible for regulating appetite. This should keep you from asking for more food, but in the case of obesity, leptin may not do its job properly. Due to the hypothalamus, the brain does not feel that the body is well nourished and constantly wants more food, as the brain somehow believes that the body is undernourished. This condition is called leptin resistance.

Build Muscle Mass

When people say they want to lose weight, they are definitely referring to fat loss and not muscle. Fat is lighter than muscle, but we all want to have an optimal BMI, right? There is a myth that a certain amount of protein is needed to maintain muscle mass. Well, that's not entirely true. In the case of fasting, growth hormone reaches incredibly high levels after 72 hours of pure fasting, so you can maintain and even increase your muscle mass due to calorie deprivation. Obviously, it's not healthy to be on a very long fasting

period, but what if you find the right ingredients to eat and have the same benefits?

Obviously, when you are on a high carbohydrate diet you are not building muscle. you are actually accumulating fat.

However, the Sirtfood diet is notrich in carbohydrates. It is rich in sirtuins, a very healthy type of protein. The founders of this diet claim that you will lose seven pounds in seven days.

However, food must create the right environment to build or maintain muscle mass, and this is what this diet does. Besides, muscles are important for your mobility and prevent the development of chronic diseases such as osteoporosis or diabetes. Believe it or not, muscles can even have a psychological advantage, as they are known to fight depression. Yes, you willdefinitely feel great about yourself when you look sporty.

SIRT1 is able to maintain muscle mass even when fasting and can even increase your muscle mass. Muscles are made up of various cells, including the satellite cell, which is activated when the muscle is damaged or stressed.

If you do some weight training, basically putting pressure on the muscle, your muscles will grow because of the satellite cell. However, the satellite cell can only be activated by SIRT1. Otherwise, your muscles won't grow, develop, or regenerate properly.

To better comprehend the significance of sirtuins, particularly SIRT1, have in mind that without them your muscles are prone to inflammation and fatigue.

In fact, muscles age without sirtuin activity. Therefore, for muscles to function properly, they really need SIRT1. Muscles do not improve over time, like wine. Keep in mind that the effects of muscle aging can begin at age 25. By the time you reach 40, you have already lost 10 percent of your muscle mass and by the time you are 70, you have already lost 40 percent of your muscle mass. However, this can be prevented and reversed through the activity of sirtuin. Therefore, they can easily be considered as regulators of muscle growth and prevention.

Fight Diseases

The modern-day eating habits and lifestyle encourages the accumulation of fats and toxins (fat tissue protects the toxins), as well as the increase of blood sugar and insulin level. This is where the trouble starts, from a simple prediabetes condition to more serious diseases (it can eventually lead to cancer).

However, the antidote to many of these issues lies hidden within ourselves.

As you already know, all bodies possess sirtuin genes, and activating them is crucial to burn fat and to build a stronger and leaner body.

As it turns out, the benefits of sirtuins activity extend way beyond the fatburning process. Whether we like it or not, the lack of sirtuins can be associated with plenty of diseases and medical conditions. Naturally, activating sirtuins will have the opposite effect. For example, sirtuins can improve your heart health by protecting the muscle cells in your heart and improving the function of the heart muscle. But that's not all. Sirtuins can play a major role in improving the function of your arteries, controlling cholesterol levels, and preventing atherosclerosis.

By now, you are familiar with the effects of fasting and an LCHF diet on the insulin level, and you are probably wondering what sirtuins can do in this case. If you are suffering from diabetes, then you should know that activating sirtuins will make insulin work more effectively to do its job properly (which is regulating the blood sugar level). SIRT1 works perfectly with metformin (one of the most powerful antidiabetic drugs). As it turns out, pharmaceutical

companies are adding sirtuin activators to metformin treatments. These studies were conducted on animals, and the results were simply amazing. It was noticed that an 83 percent reduction of the metformin dose is required to achieve the same effects.

Other diets or programs are bragging about their effects on neurodegenerative diseases, like Alzheimer's disease. Well, let's think about what sirtuins do!

They send a message to the brain, helping it make the right decisions when it comes to appetite suppression. This involves enhancing the communication signals in the brain, improving cognitive function, and lowering brain inflammation. Sirtuin activation stops the tau protein aggregation and amyloid B production, some of the most damaging things in the brains of Alzheimer's patients.

The benefits of sirtuins expand to bones as well, as they encourage the production of osteoblast cells (the ones responsible for strengthening your bones) and increase their survival. In other words, sirtuin activation is very important for overall bone health.

Now, we all know that the food we eat today can even lead to cancer, as we are literally eating small portions of poison. Diets are claiming that they represent the cure for cancer in an incipient form, but at the moment, we can't say this about Sirtfoods, as there are still plenty of studies to be done on this topic. However, it is fair to say that people who eat mostly Sirtfoods have the lowest cancer rates.

Losing weight is simply not enough nowadays, as the diet you have to follow needs to have plenty of health benefits as well; otherwise, you can't stick to it in the long run. Therefore, you need to see the bigger picture and not focus on losing a lot of pounds in a very short amount of time. The less processed food you eat, the more chances you will have to experience the health benefits from your meal plan, so you don't have to see a doctor very often.

Natural ingredients have a lot of vitamins and minerals. They have a very high nutritional value. Coincidence or not, sirtuins can mostly be found in such ingredients (essentially fruits and veggies). Therefore, you will need to unleash these benefits on your body by consuming these amazing ingredients daily.

Anti-Aging Effect

Anti-aging is somehow linked to autophagy, which is an intracellular process of repairing or replacing damaged cell parts. This is rejuvenation at an intracellular level. However, a part of this response is the lysosomal degradation pathway autophagy. Now you are probably wondering what sirtuins have to do with all of these. Well, SIRT1 can activate AMPK (and the other way around), so it can be considered one of the triggers of autophagy. But I'm going to spare you all the chemical details that you can't remember. What you need to know is that autophagy rejuvenates the cell, and this process can happen in all the cells of your body. Starting from the ones of your internal organs to the ones of your skin.

There are a few ways to induce autophagy, and it obviously has a very positive effect on your health and overall lifespan. Just think of the cell as a car and autophagy is the skilled mechanic capable of fixing or replacing any broken parts in it. Obviously, the cell will have a longer life, and this extrapolates to your overall life. If your cells are functioning properly, like a Swiss mechanical clock, then you can expect increased longevity. You can't reverse aging, as there is no such cure for it, and autophagy is not "the fountain of youth." However, this process can significantly slow down aging and its effect. And the best part is that it can be activated by sirtuins, especially SIRT1.

So far, people were not aware of too many ways to trigger autophagy. Some of them were doing it the hard way through intermittent fasting. Others were trying to induce it through an LCHF diet, like the keto diet. Well, now there is an extra way to activate it, and that is through the Sirtfood diet.

Here is a list of other benefits of the Sirtfood Diet:

- Promotes fat loss, not muscle loss
- You will not regain weight after the end of the diet
- You will look better; you will feel better, and you will have more energy
- You will avoid fasting and feeling hungry
- You will not have to undergo exhausting physical exercises

This diet promotes a longer, healthier life and keeps diseases away.

The benefits of the Sirtfood Diet are many, besides obviously that of slimming. Activators of sirtuins would lead to noticeable muscle building, decreased appetite, and improved memory. Also, the Sirtfood Diet normalizes the level of sugar in the blood and can cleanse the cells from the accumulation of harmful free radicals.

Sirtfood Green Juice

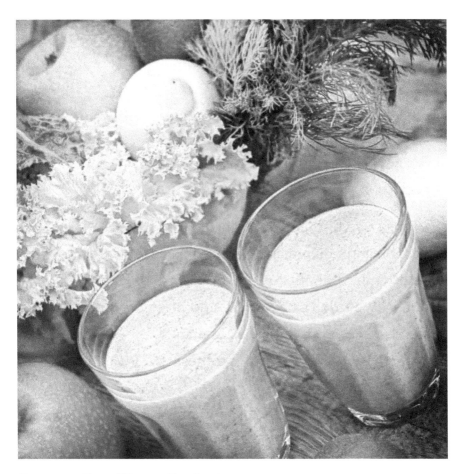

Preparation Time: 5 minutes

Cooking Time: 10 minutes

Servings: 1

Ingredients:

Recipe 1:

- 1 tablespoon parsley
- 1 stalk celery

- 1 apple
- ½ lemon

Recipe 2:

- 1 cucumber
- 1 stalk celery
- 1 apple
- 3 mint leaves

Directions:

1. Choose one of the recipes above.
2. Add all ingredients into a juicer and extract the juice according to the manufacturer's method.
3. In case you don't have one, add all the ingredients to a blender and pulse until well combined.
4. Filter the juice through a fine-mesh strainer and transfer it into a glass.
1. Top with water if needed. Serve immediately.

Nutrition: Calories 30kcal, Fat 0.4 g, Carbohydrate 4.5 g, Protein 1 g

Pancakes with Caramelized Strawberries

Preparation Time: 5 minutes

Cooking Time: 15 minutes

Servings: 2

Ingredients:

- 1 egg
- 1 ½ oz. self-raising flour
- 1 ½ oz. buckwheat flour
- 1/3 cup skimmed milk
- 1 cup strawberries
- 2 teaspoons honey

Directions:

2. Mix the flours in a bowl; add the yolk and a bit of mix in a very thick batter. Keep adding the milk bit by bit to avoid lumps.
3. In another bowl, beat the egg white until stiff and then mix it carefully to the batter.
4. Put enough batter to make a 5-inch round pancake to cook 2 minutes per side until done. Repeat until all the pancakes are ready.
5. Put strawberries and honey in a hot pan until caramelized, the put half on top of each serving.

Nutrition: Calories: 272, Fat: 4.3g, Carbohydrate: 26.8g, Protein: 23.6g

Scrambled Eggs and Red Onion

Preparation Time: 2 minutes

Cooking Time: 2 minutes

Servings: 1

Ingredients:

- 2 eggs
- 1 tablespoon Parmesan
- Salt and pepper
- ½ cup red onion
- 1 tablespoon parsley, finely chopped

Directions:

1. Put eggs and cheese with a pinch of salt and pepper and finely chopped onion in a bowl. Whisk quickly.
2. Cook the scrambled eggs in a skillet for 2 minutes, stirring continuously until done.

Nutrition: Calories: 278, Fat: 5.4g, Carbohydrate: 12.8g, Protein: 18.9g

Matcha Overnight Oats

Preparation Time: 10 minutes + overnight rest

Cooking Time: 0 minutes

Servings: 2

Ingredients:

- 2 teaspoons Chia seeds
- 3 oz. Rolled oats
- 1 teaspoon Matcha powder
- 1 teaspoon Honey
- 1 ½ cups Almond milk
- 2 pinches ground cinnamon
- 1 Apple, peeled, cored, and chopped
- 4 walnuts

Directions:

1. Place the chia seeds and the oats in a container or bowl.
2. In a different jug or bowl, add the matcha powder and one tablespoon of almond milk and whisk with a hand-held mixer until you get a smooth paste, then add the rest of the milk and mix thoroughly.
3. Pour the milk mixture over the oats, add the honey and cinnamon, and then stir well. Cover the bowl with a lid and place in the fridge overnight.
4. When you want to eat, transfer the oats to two serving bowls, then top with the walnuts, and chopped apple.

Nutrition: Calories 324, Carbs37 g, Fat14 g, Protein: 22g

Banana Blueberry Pancakes with Apple Compote and Turmeric Latte

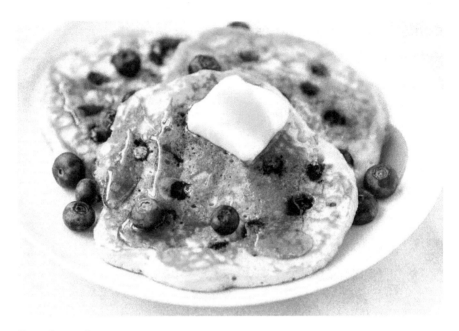

Serving: 2

Nutritional Value: 105 calories

Preparation time: 13 minutes

Cook time: 10 minutes

Total time: 23 minutes

Ingredients:

For preparing the Pancakes

- 225g blueberries
- Six bananas
- 150g oats
- Six eggs
- Two tsp baking powder

- ¼ teaspoon salt

For preparing the Apple Compote

- 1/4 teaspoon cinnamon powder
- Two apples
- One tablespoon lemon juice
- Five dates (pitted)
- salt to taste

For preparing the Turmeric Latte

- stripped ginger root
- One teaspoon turmeric powder
- Touch of dark pepper (expands ingestion)
- One teaspoon cinnamon powder
- Three cups of coconut milk
- One teaspoon crude nectar
- Touch of cayenne pepper (discretionary)

Instructions:

1. Put the oats in a rapid blender and let it grind for one moment or until an oat flour has framed. You should ensure that your blender is dry before doing this, or probably everything will get spongy.
2. Presently include the bananas, eggs, heating powder and salt to the blender and grind for 2 minutes until a smooth mixture structures.

3. Move the blend to an enormous bowl and overlay in the blueberries. Leave to rest for 10 mins while the baking powder actuates.

4. To make your cakes, include a bit of margarine to your skillet on a medium-high stove. Include a couple of spoons of the blueberry cake blend and fry for until pleasantly brilliant on the base side. Hurl the flapjack to sear the opposite side.

5. Remove the center and flat cleave your apples.

6. Pop everything in a food processor, along with two tablespoons of water and a touch of salt. Grind it to shape your stout apple compote.

7. Mix all the things in a rapid blender until smooth.

8. Fill it in a little container and warm for 4 minutes over a medium stove until hot yet not bubbling.

9. Your pancakes are ready to be served along with your latte.

Chocolate and Coffee Mousse

Serving: 8

Nutritional Value: 242 calories

Preparation time: 4 hours

Cook time: 15 minutes

Total time: 4 hours and 15 minutes

Ingredients:

- Cinnamon 1/2 tsp
- 300 ml of Almond milk
- Cocoa powder 2 tbsp
- Espresso 200 ml
- Gelatin powder 1 tbsp
- Coconut yogurt 300 g
- Maple syrup 2 tbsp
- Chocolate unadulterated 200 g

Instructions:

1. Join the almond milk and espresso in a pan and sprinkle the gelatin over it. Let it be for 5 minutes.
2. Mix the blend well and bring to bubble quickly. At that point, quickly remove the container from the stove.
3. Mix the maple syrup, cinnamon, and the dim chocolate into the hot fluid. Keep on blending until the chocolate has totally dissolved and has been assimilated into the blend.
4. Pour it in enriching pastry glasses and let it set in the refrigerator for approximately 4 hours.

5. Prior to serving, decorate with a spoon of coconut yogurt and residue with cocoa.
6. Your dish is ready to be served.

Peanut Butter Cookie Bars

Serving: 16

Nutritional Value: 350 calories

Preparation time: 40 minutes

Total time: 40 minutes

Ingredients:

- Two delicate Medjool dates
- ¼ cup in addition to 1 tablespoon maple syrup
- Two teaspoons vanilla concentrate
- Piling ½ teaspoon ocean salt
- 2½ cups almond flour
- Two tablespoons water
- ¼ cup in addition to 1 tablespoon dissolved coconut oil
- 2½ tablespoons maca powder, discretionary
- One cup of chocolate chips
- 1½ cups pecans
- Two tablespoons cacao or cocoa powder
- ¼ teaspoon ocean salt
- Flaky ocean salt for sprinkling on top, discretionary
- ½ cup in addition to 2 tablespoons smooth nutty spread

Instructions:

1. Place a heating container with material paper.

2. In an enormous bowl, mix together the nutty spread, coconut oil, maple syrup, vanilla, and salt until joined. Include the almond flour and maca if you utilize and mix to consolidate (the blend will be thick). Crease in the chocolate chips and press into the skillet.
1. Place it in the cooler with the goal that it solidifies a piece while making the following layer.
2. In a little food processor, beat the pecans, cacao powder, and ocean salt until the pecans are all around grinded. Add the dates and beat to join, including two tablespoons water if the sharp edge stalls out.
3. Keep doing the procedure until smooth. At that point, spread onto the treated layer. Sprinkle with ocean salt whenever wanted. Freeze for 30. Remove it from the container and cut it into bars. Store the remaining bars in the refrigerator.
4. Your sweet dish is ready to be eaten.

Chocolate Orange Cheesecake

Serving: 8

Nutritional Value: 374 calories

Preparation time: 30 minutes

Cook time: 2 hours

Total time: 2 hours 30 minutes

Ingredients:

- 200 g stomach related bread rolls
- 40 g margarine
- One tsp orange concentrate
- Orange sprinkles
- 250 g cream cheddar
- 120 g caster sugar
- 175 g milk chocolate
- 30 ml (32g) dual cream
- 20 g cocoa powder
- 150 ml (159g) twofold cream
- 50 g cream cheddar
- 25 g caster sugar
- 35 g white chocolate
- ¼ tsp orange concentrate
- Six cuts Chocolate Orange

Instructions:

1. Line the base of a round free bottomed tin with greaseproof paper or a reusable preparing liner.

2. Smash the rolls. Soften your margarine and blend it in with the squashed rolls. Combine the squashed bread rolls and liquefied spread. Put the bread blend into the readied tin and utilize the rear of a spoon to push it level. Put the tin into the cooler to chill while you make the cheesecake mixture.

To make the mixture of cheesecake:

1. Dissolve the milk chocolate, Put aside to cool.
2. Beat together the cream cheddar and caster sugar
3. In an alternate bowl, whisk the double cream until it shapes delicate pinnacles. Gradually include the liquefied chocolate and beat in. Filter in the cocoa powder and blend well until consolidated. Include the cream cheddar blend and orange concentrate and overlap together until everything is completely consolidated.
4. Remove the tin from the cooler and include the cheesecake blend. Utilize a little palette blade or the rear of a spoon to smooth the top (you'll have to push it down to maintain a strategic distance from air rises before smoothing).
5. Refrigerate the cheesecake.

Preparing the topping of chocolate:

1. Liquefy the white chocolate (35g). Put aside to cool.
2. Beat together the cream cheddar (50g) and caster sugar (25g).

3. In an alternate bowl, whisk the double cream (30ml) until it shapes delicate pinnacles. Gradually include the softened white chocolate and beat in. Include the cream cheddar blend and orange concentrate (¼ tsp) and overlap together until everything is completely consolidated.

4. Embellish the cheesecake

5. Take out the cheesecake from the cooler. Fit it in a channeling sack with a huge star spout. Include the white chocolate orange cheesecake blend into the funneling bag. Channel out eight whirls around the edge of the cheesecake.

6. Refrigerate to permit the cheesecake to set. Your cake is ready to be served.

7. Not long before serving, include a cut of chocolate orange on each twirl of white chocolate cheesecake. At that point, including some orange sprinkles.

8. You can follow all these amazing recipes mentioned in this chapter and make your diet days one of the amazing ones you have yet had. Have a healthy and happy life.

Celery Juice

Preparation Time: 10 minutes

Servings: 2

Ingredients:

- 8 celery stalks with leaves
- 2 tbsp. fresh ginger, peeled
- 1 lemon, peeled
- ½ cup filtered water
- Pinch of salt

Directions:

1. Add all the ingredients in a juicer and extract the juice according to the manufacturer's method.
2. If you don't have one, add all the ingredients to a blender and blend until well blended.
3. Strain the juice through a fine mesh strainer and transfer to two glasses.
4. Serve immediately.

Nutrition Facts: Calories 32kcal, Fat 0.5 g, Carbohydrate 6.5 g, Protein 1 g

Fruit and crunchy nut yogurt

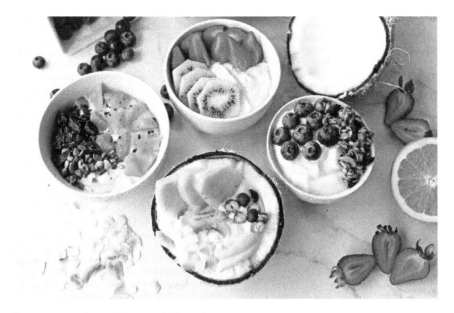

Preparation Time: 15 minutes

Servings: 1

Ingredients:

- 100g (3½ oz) plain Greek yogurt
- 50g (2oz) strawberries, chopped
- 6 walnut halves, chopped
- A sprinkling of cocoa powder

Directions

1. Stir half of the chopped strawberries into the yogurt.
2. Using a glass, place a layer of yogurt with a sprinkling of strawberries and walnuts, followed by another layer of the same until you reach the top of the glass.

3. Garnish with walnuts pieces and a dusting of cocoa powder.

Nutrition: calories 327, fat 5, fiber 11.5, carbs 11.1, protein 5.3

Banana and cinnamon oatmeals

Preparation Time: 5 minutes

Cooking Time: 5 minutes.

Servings: 6

Ingredients:

- 2 cup quick-cooking oats
- 4 cup fat-free milk
- 1 tsp. ground cinnamon
- 2 chopped large ripe banana
- 4 tsp brown sugar
- Extra ground cinnamon

Directions:

1. Place milk in a skillet and bring to boil. Add oats and cook over medium heat until thickened, for two to four minutes.
2. Stir intermittently.
3. Add cinnamon, brown sugar, and banana and stir to combine.
4. If you want, serve with the extra cinnamon and milk. Enjoy!

Nutrition: calories 217, fat 5.5, fiber 14.5, carbs 1.1, protein 5.3

Healthy bagels

Preparation Time: 15 minutes

Cooking Time: 60 minutes.

Servings: 8

Ingredients:

- 1 ½ cup warm water
- 1 ¼ cup bread flour
- 2 tbsp honey
- 2 cup whole wheat flour
- 2 tsp yeast
- 1 ½ tbsp extra virgin olive oil
- 1 tbsp vinegar

Directions

1. In a bread machine, mix all ingredients, and then process on dough cycle.
2. Once done, create 8 pieces shaped like a flattened ball.
3. Make a hole in the center of each ball using your thumb then create a donut shape.
4. In a greased baking sheet, place donut-shaped dough then cover and let it rise about ½ hour.
5. Prepare about 2 inches of water to boil in a large pan.
6. In boiling water, drop one at a time the bagels and boil for 1 minute, then turn them once.

7. Remove them and return them to the baking sheet and bake at 350oF for about 20 to 25 minutes until golden brown.

Nutrition: calories 327, fat 5, fiber 11.5, carbs 11.1, protein 5.3

Cranberry and orange cereals

Preparation Time: 5 minutes

Cooking Time: 2 minutes.

Servings: 1

Ingredients:

- ½ cup of water
- ½ cup of orange juice
- 1/3 cup of oat bran
- ¼ cup of dried cranberries
- Sugar
- Milk

Directions

1. In a bowl, combine all ingredients.
2. For about 2 minutes, microwave the bowl then serve with sugar and milk.

Nutrition: calories 327, fat 5, fiber 1.5, carbs 11.1, protein 5.3

Vegan rice pudding

Preparation Time: 5 minutes

Cooking Time: 20 minutes.

Servings: 8

Ingredients:

- ½ tsp ground cinnamon
- 1 cup rinsed basmati
- 1/8 tsp ground cardamom
- ¼ cup sugar
- 1/8 tsp pure almond extract
- 1-quart vanilla nondairy milk
- 1 tsp pure vanilla extract

Directions

1. Measure all of the ingredients into a saucepan and stir well to combine.
2. Bring to a boil over medium-high heat.
3. Remove from heat and cool.
4. Serve sprinkled with additional ground cinnamon if desired.

Nutrition: calories 327, fat 2, fiber 1.5, carbs 1.1, protein 2.3

Cinnamon scented quinoa breakfast

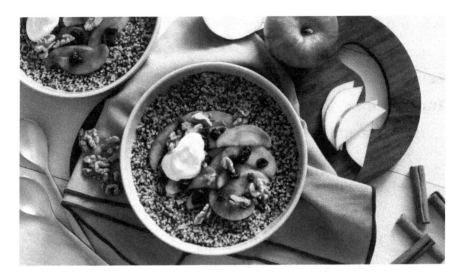

Preparation Time: 20 minutes

Cooking Time: 10 minutes.

Servings: 4

Ingredients:

- Chopped walnuts
- 1 ½ cup water
- Maple syrup
- 2 cinnamon sticks
- 1 cup quinoa

Directions.

1. When washing quinoa, rub grains and allow them to settle before you pour off the water.
2. Use a large fine-mesh sieve to drain the quinoa.
3. Prepare your pressure cooker with a trivet and steaming basket.

4. Place the quinoa and the cinnamon sticks in the basket and pour the water.
5. Close and lock the lid.
6. Cook at high pressure for 6 minutes. When the cooking time is up, release the pressure using the quick-release method.
7. Fluff the quinoa with a fork and remove the cinnamon sticks. Divide the cooked quinoa among serving bowls and top with maple syrup and chopped walnuts.

Nutrition: calories 127, fat 2, fiber 1, carbs 1, protein 5.3

Oatmeal banana pancakes with walnuts

Preparation Time: 15 minutes

Cooking Time: 15 minutes.

Servings: 8

Ingredients:

- 1 finely diced firm banana
- 1 cup whole wheat pancake mix
- 1/8 cup chopped walnuts
- ¼ cup old-fashioned oats

Directions

1. Make the pancake mix according to the directions on the package.
2. Add walnuts, oats, and chopped banana.
3. Coat a griddle with cooking spray.
4. Add about ¼ cup of the pancake batter onto the griddle when hot.
5. Turn pancake over when bubbles form on top. Cook until golden brown.
6. Serve immediately.

Nutrition: calories 178, fat 2, fiber 7, carbs 1, protein 4

Cheesy baked eggs

Preparation Time: 15 minutes

Cooking Time: 30 hours

Servings: 4

Ingredients:

- 4 large eggs
- 75g (3oz) cheese, grated
- 25g (1oz) fresh rocket (arugula) leaves, finely chopped
- 1 tablespoon parsley
- ½ teaspoon ground turmeric
- 1 tablespoon olive oil

Directions

1. Grease each ramekin dish with a little olive oil.
2. Divide the rocket (arugula) between the ramekin dishes then break an egg into each one.
3. Sprinkle a little parsley and turmeric on top then sprinkle on the cheese.
4. Place the ramekins in a preheated oven at 220C/425F for 15 minutes, until the eggs are set and the cheese is bubbling.

Nutrition: calories 127, fat 2, fiber 11.5, carbs 1.1, protein 5.3

LUNCH
Green Beans with Vegan Bacon

Preparation Time: 15 minutes

Cooking Time: 20 minutes

Servings: 8

Ingredients:

- 2 slices of vegan bacon, chopped
- 1 shallot, chopped
- 24 oz. green beans
- Salt and pepper to taste
- ½ teaspoon smoked paprika
- 1 teaspoon lemon juice
- 2 teaspoons vinegar

Directions:

1. Preheat your oven to 450 degrees F.
2. Add the bacon to the baking pan and roast for 5 minutes.
3. Stir in the shallot and beans.
4. Season it with salt, pepper, and paprika.
5. Roast for 10 minutes.
6. Drizzle with lemon juice and vinegar.
7. Roast for another 2 minutes.

Nutrition:

Calories: 49,Fat: 1.2g,Saturated fat: 0.4g,Cholesterol: 3mg,Potassium: 249mg,Carbohydrates: 8.1g,Fiber: 3g,Sugar: 4g,Protein: 2.9g

Chicken Breakfast Skillet

Preparation Time: 30 minutes

Cooking Time: 30 minutes

Servings: 2

Ingredients:

- 1 chicken breast
- 3 ounces ground sausage
- 2 eggs
- 3 slices bacon
- ½ teaspoon garlic powder
- ½ teaspoon ground black pepper

Directions:

1. Chop the bacon and chicken breast into pieces roughly one inch in size. Add the bacon to a skillet over medium heat and cook for two minutes, stirring frequently. Once the bacon grease has begun to accumulate in the pan, stir in the diced chicken and ground or crumbled sausage.

2. Add garlic powder and pepper to the meat in the skillet. Brown the meat over medium-high heat for about six to eight minutes.

3. Reduce heat to medium. On opposite sides of the pan, clear two pockets of space for the eggs. Crack the eggs into the skillet and break the yolks apart. Cover the skillet

and allow cooking so that the egg whites are firm about 10 minutes. Uncover and scoop onto a plate to serve.

Nutrition:

Calories: 341, Fat: 19 g, Sodium: 631 mg, Carbohydrates: 1 g,Fiber: 0 g, Sugar: 1 g, Protein: 36 g

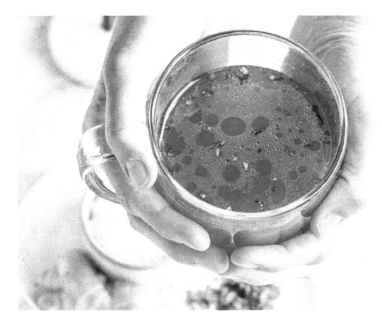

Preparation Time: 15 minutes

Cooking Time: 24 hours

Servings: 16

Ingredients:

- 3 pounds of assorted animal bones, with marrow
- 1 gallon of water
- 3 tablespoons salt
- 2 tablespoons ground black pepper

Directions:

1. Add assorted bones to a slow cooker. Pour in the water and season with salt and pepper. Turn the slow cooker to high.

2. Bring the water inside the slow cooker to a boil. This may take up to 20 minutes due to a large amount of water. Then reduce the temperature settings to low and allow to simmer for up to 24 hours.

1. Letting the bone broth cook for this long gives you a more nutritious and tastier product. You do not need to stir the broth during this time. If necessary, add more water around the 12-hour mark if you notice the water level has dropped far below the top of the bones.

2. Shut off the heat and let the broth cool. Strain into a large stockpot or other container and discard the remains of the bones. Enjoy hot or allow cooling completely before packaging for refrigeration or freezing. The bone broth will solidify in the fridge, so simply reheat leftovers.

Nutrition:

Calories: 56,Fat: 2 g,Sodium: 480 mg,Carbohydrates: 0 g,Fiber: 0 g,Sugar: 0 g,Protein: 9 g

Preparation Time: 30 minutes

Cooking Time: 10 minutes

Servings: 2

Ingredients:

- 1 teaspoon tomato puree
- 1-star anise, crushed (or 1/4 teaspoon anise)
- A small handful (10 g) of parsley, finely chopped stalks
- A small handful of coriander (10 g), finely chopped stalks
- Juice from 1/2 lime
- 500 ml chicken broth, fresh or made from 1 cube
- 1/2 carrot, peeled and cut into matches
- 50 g broccoli, cut into small roses
- 50 g bean sprouts
- 100 g raw tiger prawns
- 100 g hard tofu, chopped
- 50 g rice noodles, cooked according to the instructions on the packaging
- 50g of boiled water chestnuts, drained
- 20g chopped ginger sushi
- 1 tablespoon of good quality miso paste

Directions:

1. Place in a large saucepan the tomato purée, star anise, parsley stalks, coriander stalks, lime juice, and chicken stock and bring 10 minutes to a simmer.
2. Stir in the cabbage, broccoli, prawns, tofu, noodles, and water chestnuts, and cook gently until the prawns are finished. Remove from heat and whisk in the ginger sushi and the paste miso.
3. Serve sprinkled with the leaves of the parsley and coriander.

Nutrition:

Calories: 253 Cal, Fat: 7.35 g, Carbohydrates: 29.99 g, Protein: 19.39, Fiber: 6 g

Salmon Fritters

Preparation Time: 10 minutes

Cooking Time: 20 minutes

Servings: 2

Ingredients:

- 6 oz. salmon, canned
- 1 tablespoon flour
- 1 clove garlic, crushed
- ½ red onion, finely chopped
- 2 eggs
- 2 teaspoons olive oil
- Salt and pepper to taste
- 2 cups arugula

Directions:

1. Separate egg whites from yolks and beat them until very stiff. In a separate bowl mix salmon, flour, salt, pepper, onion, garlic, onion, and yolks.
2. Add egg whites and slowly mix them together. Heat a pan on mediumhigh.
1. Add 1teaspoon oil and when hot form salmon fritters with a spoon.
2. Cook until brown (around 4 minutes per side) and serve with arugula salad seasoned with salt, pepper, and 1 teaspoon olive oil.

Nutrition: Calories: 320 Carbs: 18g Fat: 7g Protein: 27g

Mince Stuffed Eggplants

Preparation Time: 10 minutes

Cooking Time: 70 minutes

Servings: 6

Ingredients:

- 4 oz. lean mince
- 6 large eggplants
- 1 egg
- 3 tablespoon dry red wine
- ½ cup cheddar, grated
- Salt and pepper, to taste
- 1 red onion
- 2 teaspoons olive oil
- 2 tablespoons tomato sauce
- 2 tablespoons parsley

Directions:

1. Preheat oven to 350°F. Meanwhile, slice eggplants in 2 and scoop out the center part, leaving ½ inch of meat. . Place eggplants in a microwavable dish with about ½" of water in the bottom.
2. Microwave on high for 4 minutes. In a saucepan, fry mince with onion for 5 minutes.
3. Add wine and let evaporate.
4. Add tomato sauce, salt, pepper, eggplant meat and cook for around 20 minutes until done.

5. Combine, mince sauce, cheese, egg, parsley, salt, and pepper in a large bowl and mix well. Pack firmly into eggplants.

6. Return eggplants to the dish you first microwaved them in and bake for 25 to 30 minutes, or until lightly browned on top.

Nutrition: Calories: 350 Carbs: 22g Fat: 10g Protein: 17g

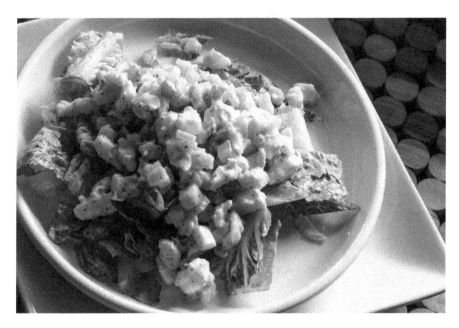

Easy Shrimp Salad

Preparation Time: 5 minutes

Cooking Time: 0 minutes

Servings: 2

Ingredients:

- 2 cups red endive, finely sliced
- 1 cup cherry tomatoes, halved
- 1 teaspoon of EVO oil
- 1 tablespoon parsley, chopped
- 3 oz. celery, sliced
- 6 walnuts, chopped
- 2 oz. red onion-sliced
- 1 cup yellow pepper, cubed
- ½ lemon, juiced
- 6 oz. steamed shrimps

Directions:

1. Put red endive on a large plate. Evenly distribute on top finely sliced onion, yellow pepper, cherry tomatoes walnuts, celery, and parsley.
2. Mix oil, lemon juice with a pinch of salt and pepper and distribute the dressing on top.

Nutrition: Calories: 353, Fat: 4.8g, Carbohydrate: 28.1g, Protein: 28.3g

Red Onion Frittata with Chili Grilled Zucchini

Preparation Time: 5 minutes

Cooking Time: 30 minutes

Servings: 2

Ingredients:

- 1 ½ cups red onion, finely sliced
- 3 eggs
- 3 oz. cheddar cheese
- 2 tablespoons milk
- 2 zucchini
- 2 tablespoons oil
- 1 clove garlic, crushed
- ½ chili, finely sliced
- 1 teaspoon white vinegar
- Salt and pepper to taste

Directions:

1. Heat the oven to 350°F. Cut the zucchini into thin slices; grill them and set them aside.
2. Add 3 eggs, shredded cheddar cheese, milk, salt, pepper, whisk well and pour in a silicone baking tray and cook 25-30 minutes in the oven.
3. Mix garlic, oil, salt, pepper, and vinegar and pour the dressing on the zucchini. Serve the frittata alongside the zucchini.

Nutrition: Calories: 359, Fat: 7.8g, Carbohydrate: 18.1g, Protein: 21.3g

Garlic Chicken Burgers

Preparation Time: 10 minutes

Cooking Time: 10 minutes

Servings: 2

Ingredients:

- 8 oz. chicken mince
- ¼ red onion, finely chopped
- 1 clove garlic, crushed
- 1 handful of parsley, finely chopped
- 1 cup arugula
- ½ orange, chopped
- 1 cup cherry tomatoes
- 3 teaspoons EVO oil

Directions:

1. Put chicken mince, onion, garlic, parsley, salt pepper in a bowl and mix well. Form 2 patties and let rest 5 minutes.
2. Heat a pan with olive oil and when very hot cook 3 minutes per part.
3. They are also very good when grilled, if you opt for grilling; just brush the patties with a bit of oil right before cooking.
4. Put the arugula on two plates; add cherry tomatoes and orange on top, dress with salt and the remaining olive oil. Put the patties on top and serve.

Nutrition: Calories: 353, Fat: 4.8g, Carbohydrate: 28.1g, Protein: 28.3g

Turmeric Turkey Breast with Cauliflower Rice

Preparation Time: 5 minutes

Cooking Time: 25 minutes

Servings: 2

Ingredients:

- 2 cups cauliflower, grated
- 8 oz. turkey breast, cut into slices
- 2 teaspoons ground turmeric
- 1/2 pepper, chopped
- 1/2 red onion, sliced
- 2 teaspoons EVO oil
- 1 large tomato
- 1 clove garlic, crushed
- 1 cup milk, skimmed
- 2 teaspoons buckwheat flour
- 1 oz. parsley, finely chopped

Directions:

1. Coat turkey slices with flour.
2. Heat a pan on medium-high with half the oil and when hot add the turkey.
3. Let the meat color on all sides, then add milk, salt, pepper, 1 teaspoon turmeric. Cook 10 minutes until the turkey is soft and the sauce has become creamy.

4. In a different pan, add the remaining oil and heat on medium heat. Add pepper, onion, and tomato, 1 teaspoon turmeric and let cook 3 minutes.
5. Add the cauliflower and cook for another 2 minutes. Add salt, pepper and let rest 2 minutes.
6. Serve the turkey with the cauliflower rice.

Nutrition: Calories 107 Total Fat 2.9 g Total Carbs 20.6 g Protein 2.1 g

Mustard Salmon with Baby Carrots

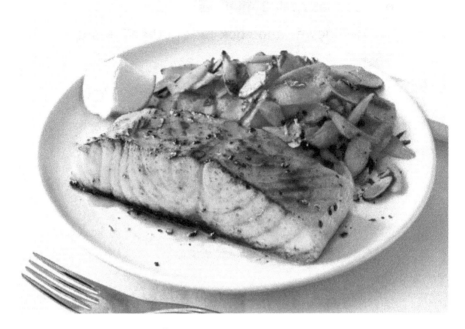

Preparation Time: 10 minutes

Cooking Time: 40 minutes

Servings: 2

Ingredients:

- 8 oz. salmon fillet
- 2 tablespoon mustard
- 1 tablespoon white vinegar
- 1 teaspoon parsley, finely chopped
- 2 cups baby carrots
- 4 oz. buckwheat
- 2 teaspoons EVO oil
- Salt and pepper to taste

Directions:

1. Heat the oven to 400°F.
2. Boil the buckwheat in salted water for 25 minutes then drain. Dress with 1 teaspoon olive oil. Set aside. Put the salmon over aluminum foil.
3. Mix mustard and vinegar in a small bowl and brush the mixture over the salmon, close the foil in a packet. Cook in the oven for 35 minutes.
4. While the salmon is cooking, steam baby carrots for 6 minutes then put them in a pan on medium heat with 1teaspoon olive oil, salt, and pepper until light brown.
5. Serve the salmon with baby carrots and buckwheat on the side.

Nutrition: Calories 314, Fat 9.1g, Protein 41.5g, Carbohydrate 15.7g

Turmeric Couscous with Edamame Beans

Preparation Time: 10 minutes

Cooking Time: 15 minutes

Servings: 2

Ingredients:

- ½ yellow pepper, cubed
- ½ red pepper, cubed
- 1 tablespoon turmeric
- ½ cup red onion, finely sliced
- ¼ cup cherry tomatoes, chopped
- 2 tablespoon parsley, finely chopped
- 5 oz. couscous
- 2 teaspoons EVO oil
- ½ eggplant
- 1 ½ edamame beans

Directions:

1. Steam edamame for 5 minutes and set aside. Add 6 oz. salted boiling water to couscous and let rest until it absorbs the water.
2. In the meantime, heat a pan on medium-high heat.
3. Add oil, eggplant, peppers, onion and tomatoes, turmeric, salt, and pepper. Cook for 5 minutes on high heat.
4. Add the couscous and edamame.
5. Garnish with fresh parsley and serve.

Nutrition: Calories 342, Carbs 15 g, Fat 5 g, Protein: 32g

Mozzarella Cauliflower Bars

Preparation Time: 10 minutes

Cooking Time: 40 minutes

Servings: 12

Ingredients:

- 1 big cauliflower head, riced
- ½ cup low-fat mozzarella cheese, shredded
- ¼ cup egg whites
- 1 teaspoon Italian seasoning
- Black pepper to the taste

Directions:

1. Spread the cauliflower rice on a lined baking sheet, cook in the oven at 375 degrees F for 20 minutes, transfer to a bowl, add black pepper, cheese, seasoning, and egg whites, stir well, spread into a rectangle pan, and press well on the bottom.
2. Introduce in the oven at 375 degrees F, bake for 20 minutes, cut into 12 bars, and serve as a snack.

Nutrition:

Calories 140, Fat 1, Fiber 3, Carbs 6, Protein 6

DINNER
Shrimp and Pineapple Salsa

Preparation Time: 10 minutes

Cooking Time: 40 minutes

Servings: 4

Ingredients:

- 1-pound large shrimp, peeled and deveined
- 20 ounces canned pineapple chunks
- 1 tablespoon garlic powder
- 1 cup red bell peppers, chopped
- Black pepper to the taste

Directions:

1. Place shrimp in a baking dish, add pineapple, garlic, bell peppers, and black pepper, toss a bit, introduce in the oven.
2. Bake at 375 degrees F for 40 minutes, divide into small bowls and serve cold.

Nutrition:

Calories 170, Fat 5, Fiber 4, Carbs 15, Protein 11

Vegetarian Parmesan Risotto

Preparation Time: 65 minutes

Cooking Time: 50 minutes

Servings: 5

Ingredients:

- 2 cups Arborio rice
- ½ cup plain white rice
- 1 cup veggie stock
- 1 cup water
- 6-8 ounces Parmesan cheese, grated
- 1 onion, chopped
- 1 tablespoon butter
- Salt and black pepper to taste

Directions:

1. Prepare a water bath and place Sous Vide in it. Set to 185 F. Melt the butter in a saucepan over medium heat.
2. Add onions, rice, and spices, and cook for a few minutes. Transfer to a vacuum-sealable bag. Release air by the water displacement method, seal and submerge the bag in a water bath. Set the timer for 50 minutes.
3. Once the timer has stopped, remove the bag and stir in the Parmesan cheese.

Nutrition:

Calories: 433, Total Fat: 10.5g, Cholesterol: 30mg, Total Carbs: 68.1g, Fiber: 2.6g, Sugars: 1.3g, Protein: 16.6g

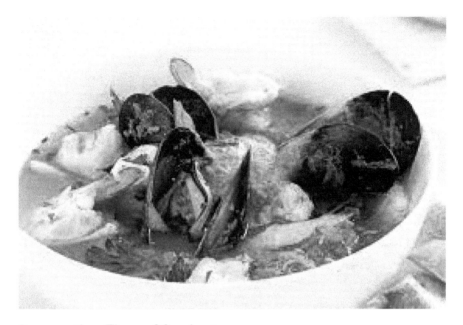

Preparation Time: 20 minutes

Cooking Time: 2 hours and 30 minutes

Servings: 6

Ingredients:

- 1 ½ lb clams (cleaned, rinsed)
- 1 ½ lbs grouper
- ½ lb octopus
- 1 tablespoon
- Parsley (fresh)
- 3 teaspoons olive oil
- 2 garlic cloves
- Black pepper (to taste)
- Salt (to taste)

- 1 red bell pepper (chopped)
- 1 green bell pepper (chopped)
- 2 jalapeno peppers (minced)
- 10 ounces tomatoes (canned)
- ½ teaspoon dill weed (dried)
- ½ teaspoon lemon rind (freshly grated is better)
- 1 teaspoon rosemary (dried)
- ½ teaspoon basil (dried)
- 3 cups water

Directions:

1. Grab your sous vide water bath and preheat it to 140 degrees F.
2. You could use your ping pong balls to regulate the temperature even better.
3. Season your clams to your taste with salt and pepper.
4. Put the clams, garlic, parsley, and a teaspoon of olive oil into a Ziploc bag. Seal the bag nice and tight.
5. Submerge the Ziploc bag into your sous vide water bath, making sure it's below the ping pong balls. Allow this to cook for 10 minutes, then you can take it out.
6. Now, preheat your water bath to 149 degrees F. Leave the ping pong balls if you've got them in there!
7. Now, you're going to season your octopus with pepper and salt to taste.
8. After seasoning the octopus, put it in a Ziploc bag. Add a teaspoon of olive oil to the bag, and then seal it nice and

tight. Put it in the sous vide water bath and allow it to cook for an hour and fifty minutes. Take it out when the time elapses.

9. Now, preheat your sous vide water bath to 137 degrees F.

10.Grab another Ziploc bag, and then add in the rest of the olive oil, as well as the peppers, grouper, tomatoes, and seasonings.

11.Submerge the Ziploc bag into your sous vide water bath and all it to cook for just 20 minutes.

12.Once done, take all the ingredients out of their Ziploc bags, and then move them to a stockpot on medium-high heat.

13.Add in three cups of water, and then allow your stew to simmer, until it's all nicely heated up.

14.Ladle this glorious stew into your serving bowls.

Nutrition:

Calories 273, Protein: 45.1g, Fat: 5.1g, Carbs: 9.3g, Sugars: 2.7g

Coconut Cod Stew

Preparation Time: 30 minutes

Cooking Time: 30 minutes

Servings: 6

Ingredients:

- 2 lbs. fresh cod (cut into fillets
- Salt and freshly ground black pepper, to taste
- 1 can (15 ounces coconut milk, divided)
- 1 tablespoon olive oil
- 1 sweet onion (julienned)
- 1 red bell pepper (julienned)
- 4 garlic cloves (minced)
- 1 can (15 ounces) crushed tomatoes
- 1 teaspoon fish sauce
- 1 teaspoon lime juice
- Sriracha hot sauce, to taste
- 2 tablespoon chopped fresh cilantro leaves

Directions:

1. Preheat water to 130°F in a sous vide cooker or with an immersion circulator.
2. Season cod fillets with salt and pepper and vacuum-seal with ¼ cup coconut milk in a sous vide bag (or use a plastic zip-top freezer bag, removing as much air as possible from the bag before sealing). Submerge bag in water and cook for 30 minutes.

3. Immediately begin preparing the sauce. Heat olive oil in a nonstick skillet over medium-high heat and sauté onion and bell pepper until softened, 3 to 4 minutes, stirring frequently. Add garlic and sauté about 1 minute more, stirring constantly.

4. Add undrained tomatoes, fish sauce, lime juice, sriracha sauce, and remaining coconut milk and stir until thoroughly combined. Season sauce to taste with salt and pepper, reduce heat to low, and simmer until the end of the cooking time for the cod, stirring occasionally.

5. Remove cod from the cooking bag, add to sauce and turn gently to coat with sauce. Let stew stand for about 5 minutes. Garnish the stew with cilantro leaves to serve. Enjoy!

Nutrition:

Calories: 400, Total Fat: 18g, Saturated Fat: 13g, Protein: 40g, Carbs: 23g, Fiber: 5g, Sugar: 2g

Cornish Hen Stew

Preparation Time: 20 minutes

Cooking Time: 4 hours

Servings: 4

Ingredients:

- 2 tablespoons coconut oil
- 4 medium shallots, smashed and peeled
- 3 cloves garlic, smashed and peeled
- 2 lemongrass stalks, roughly chopped
- Piece fresh ginger, thinly sliced
- 5 dried red Thai chilies
- 2 teaspoons dried green peppercorns, coarsely ground
- 1 teaspoon ground turmeric cups water
- 2 whole Cornish game hens
- 1/2 cup chopped cilantro
- 2 scallions, coarsely chopped
- 2 tablespoons Asian fish sauce
- 1 teaspoon finely grated lime zest
- Kosher salt and freshly ground black pepper

Directions:

1. Set your sous to vide machine to 150°F.
2. In a large skillet, melt the coconut oil over medium heat. When hot, add the shallots, garlic, lemongrass, ginger, chilies, peppercorns, and turmeric. Cook, stirring

occasionally until shallots begin to soften, about 5 minutes.

3. Add the water to the skillet and stir, making sure to scrape the bottom of the pan. Carefully transfer to a large ziplock or vacuum-seal bag. Add the game hens to the bag and then seal using the water displacement method. Place the bag in the water bath and set the timer for 4 hours.

4. When ready, remove the bag from the water bath and take out the hens. Let the hen rest until cool enough to handle. Separate the legs, wings, and breast meat.

5. Add the cooking liquid to a large pot and bring it to a simmer over medium-high heat. Stir in the cilantro, scallions, fish sauce, lime juice, and game hen meat. Season to taste with salt and pepper.

Nutrition:

Calories: 82, Total Fat: 7g, Cholesterol: 0mg, Total Carbs: 5.4g, Fiber: 0.8g, Sugars: 0.3g, Protein: 0.9g

Spicy Asian Noodle Soup

Preparation Time: 10 minutes

Cooking Time: 30 minutes

Servings: 2

Ingredients:

- One packet of buckwheat noodles, prepared as directed on the
- package
- One small red onion
- 2 Celery stalks washed and chopped
- One piece of ginger, diced
- One garlic clove, chopped
- 1 cup arugula
- ¼ cup basil leaves, clean, dry, then chop
- ¼ cup walnuts
- 1 A teaspoon of sesame seeds
- 2 Tablespoons of black currant
- ½ chili
- 5 cups chicken or vegetable broth
- ½ lime juice
- One teaspoon EVO oil
- One tablespoon soya sauce

Directions:

1. Cook the pasta according to the instructions and set aside.

2. Sauté all the vegetables, ginger, garlic, chili, and nuts in a pan over deficient heat for about 10 minutes, add the broth and simmer for another 5 minutes. Cut the pasta (roughly) so that it is small enough to be eaten comfortably in a soup.
3. Add this to the broth, add the sesame seeds and lime juice, and remove from the heat. Refrigerate and serve.

Nutrition:

Carbs 12 g, Dietary Fiber 0 g, Sugar 2 g, Fat2 g, Protein 0 g, Sodium 546 mg

Green Soup

Preparation Time: 55 minutes

Cooking Time: 40 minutes

Servings: 3

Ingredients:

- 4 cups vegetable stock
- 1 tablespoon olive oil
- 1 clove garlic, crushed
- 1-inch ginger, sliced
- 1 teaspoon coriander powder
- 1 large zucchini, diced
- 3 cups kale
- 2 cups broccoli, cut into florets
- 1 lime, juiced, and zested

Directions:

1. Make a water bath, place Sous Vide in it, and set to 185 F. Place the broccoli, zucchini, kale, and parsley in a vacuum-sealable bag. Release air by the water displacement method, seal, and submerge the bag in the water bath. Set the timer for 30 minutes.

2. Once the timer has stopped, remove, and unseal the bag. Add the steamed ingredients to a blender with garlic and ginger—puree to smooth.

3. Pour the green puree into a pot and add the remaining listed ingredients. Put the pot over medium heat and simmer for 10 minutes. Serve as a light dish.

Nutrition:

Calories: 129, Total Fat: 5.3g, Cholesterol: 0mg, Total Carbs: 18.9g, Fiber: 5.2g, Sugars: 4.2g, Protein: 5.8g

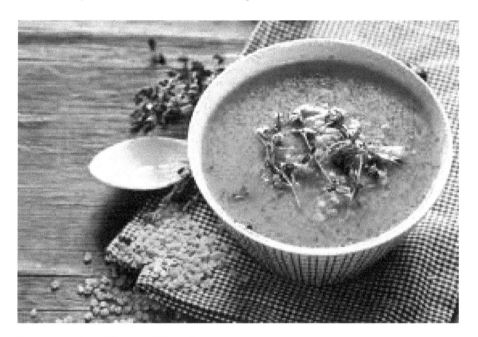

Preparation Time: 20 minutes

Cooking Time: 20 minutes

Servings: 2

Ingredients:

- 5 cups chicken or vegetable broth
- One minced chicken breast (good use for remaining chicken broths
- from other recipes!
- One small red onion
- 2 Cups of finely chopped kale
- 1 cup chopped spinach
- 1 cup lentils
- One celery stalk, chopped

- One carrot, chopped
- One little pepper or a pinch of cayenne pepper
- A pinch of salt
- One teaspoon EVO oil

Directions:

1. Cook the lentils according to the package, but take them out only a few minutes before they are cooked. Put aside.
2. Put the vegetables in a large saucepan and sauté in a little oil over medium heat. Stir until the vegetables are softer but not well cooked. Add the chicken (pre-cooked skinless chicken), add the reserved lentils, and cook for another 3 to 5 minutes. Add a pinch of salt.
3. Add the broth, simmer and simmer for 20 minutes. Stay away from heat. Serve as fresh.

Nutrition:

Calories: 467kcal, Carbohydrates: 61g, Protein: 43g, Fat: 7g, Saturated Fat: 2g, Cholesterol: 56mg, Sodium: 848mg, Fiber: 12g, Sugar: 4g

Fall Squash Cream Soup

Preparation Time: 20 minutes

Cooking Time: 2 hours

Servings: 6

Ingredients:

- ¾ cup heavy cream
- 1 winter squash, chopped
- 1 large pear
- ½ yellow onion, diced
- 3 fresh thyme sprigs
- 1 garlic clove, chopped
- 1 teaspoon ground cumin
- Salt and black pepper to taste
- 4 tablespoon crème fraîche

Directions:

1. Prepare a water bath and place the Sous Vide in it. Set to 186 F.
2. Combine the squash, pear, onion, thyme, garlic, cumin, and salt. Place it in a vacuum-sealable bag. Release air by the water displacement seal and submerge the bag in the water bath—Cook for 2 hours.
3. Once the timer has stopped, remove the bag and transfer all the contents into a blender. Puree until smooth. Add the cream and stir well. Season with salt and pepper.

Transfer the mix into serving bowls and top with some créme Fraiche. Garnish with pear chunks.

Nutrition:

Calories: 101, Total Fat: 5.8g, Cholesterol: 21mg, Total Carbs: 12.9g,Fiber: 2.3g, Sugars: 2.7g, Protein: 1.2g

Cream of Corn Soup

Preparation Time: 10 minutes

Cooking Time: 40 minutes

Servings: 4

Ingredients:

- Kernels of 4 corn ears
- 6 cups still water
- 1 cup heavy cream
- 1 tablespoon olive oil
- Salt and pepper to taste

Directions:

1. Set your cooking device to 183 degrees F.
2. Place the kernels, salt, pepper, and olive oil into the plastic bag and seal it, removing the air.
3. Set the cooking time for 25 minutes.
4. Transfer the cooked kernels with the liquid to a pot. Add the cream and still water (if needed and simmer on medium heat for about 10 minutes.
5. Blend the soup with an immersion blender, and salt and pepper if needed, and serve with chopped parsley.

CPSIA information can be obtained
at www.ICGtesting.com
Printed in the USA
LVHW081327220621
690776LV00010B/498

9 781802 920659